Table of Contents

The Intersection of Anxiety and Disability: Social Security, Accommodations, and Support

1. Introduction to Anxiety Disorders and Disability

These 15 cases serve as a catalyst for four main themes that we explore in this essay. First, our anxiety analysis reveals that anxiety can be disabling, which—in many cases—provides limited access to social security benefits. Second, although anxiety disorder-related disability presents significant limitations in the workplace and in society at large, there are few court cases and even fewer EEOC decisions that implicate anxiety as a condition requiring reasonable accommodations. Third, we demonstrate that, despite little previous case law, the myriad ways in which anxiety can interact with other disabling conditions can suggest workplace accommodations. Fourth, our essay demonstrates that heightened levels of support services are often helpful in evaluating disability petitions associated with anxiety.

Given the prevalence of anxiety and its ties to disability, we find cause to explore how anxiety is addressed—or not—within the legal framework of disability. We hope to spark a conversation about specific ways in which anxiety and disability intersect, as well as share our own lessons about 15 anxiety petitions decided through the EEOC that can offer guidance for advocates seeking accommodations for clients with disabling anxiety-related conditions.

In the United States, anxiety disorders are the most commonly reported disability, affecting over 40 million adults and 4 million children. Moreover, people with disabilities are far more likely than those without a disability to report serious psychological distress. When people with disabilities share medical records or work histories, they frequently present anxiety conditions as part of the disabling constellation.

Anxiety and Disability

2. Legal Framework: Anxiety as a Disability

SSA's list of impairments, or "blue book," outlines the criteria for a mental disorder that is so severe it prevents an adult from working, or a child from obtaining an education and preparing for work. Within the adult mental disorders section of the "blue book," the first domain of impairment that impacts anxiety is 12.00 - "Mental Disorders - Neurocognitive disorders (12.02), schizophrenia spectrum and other psychotic disorders (12.03), depressive, bipolar and related disorders (12.04), intellectual disorder (12.05), anxiety and obsessive-compulsive disorders (12.06), somatic symptom and related disorders (12.07), personality and impulse-control disorders (12.08), autism spectrum disorder (12.10), and neurodevelopmental disorders (12.11). In some cases, the guidelines provide as follows. If you have medical evidence of an anxiety-related disorder and simple work-related decisions or simple work-related tasks are precluded by your condition and symptoms, then you may be eligible for disability benefits. In other cases, the guidelines may provide disability eligibility with a severe mental disorder or anxiety-related disorder alternatively impact your ability to: understand, remember, or apply information; interact with others; concentrate, persist or maintain pace; or adapt or manage oneself. Simple tasks, however, are often invoked as problematic. Thus, SSA rules provide presumptions that can operate in one's favor to demonstrate a disability because of anxiety.

Studies have long shown that anxiety can reach a level of severity where it impacts multiple areas of one's life in spite of medication and psychotherapy. However, to be eligible for services and supports, those with mental health challenges must demonstrate from a legal and policy perspective that they have a disability as defined by social security law or agency regulations. This is true whether we speak of supports and accommodations in the realm of social security benefits, mental health, or housing. Therefore, we must address the question: What is the legal framework that exists with respect to anxiety as a disability?

2.1. Defining Disability Under Social Security Law

Furthermore, in order to qualify for disability, a person must have evidence of physical or mental defects that are severe enough to prevent the performance of any substantial gainful activity. If he or she claims to be suffering from physical or mental impairments indicating an inability to work, direct medical and other evidence (subjective complaints alone are not sufficient to establish inability to work) of the existence of an impairment is required, showing the nature and severity of the impairment sufficient to prevent an individual from engaging in the most important job the person could do on a full-time basis and showing the extent of their earning capacity.

Social Security Disability benefits are only available to individuals who meet the statutory definition of disability. Under Social Security Law, an individual who is unable to engage in any substantial gainful activity due to a medically determinable physical or mental impairment, which can be expected to result in death or has lasted or is expected to last for a continuous period of not less than 12 months, is treated as being disabled. Impairments that are classified do not require further inquiry to establish a likelihood of disability, other than considering the vocational factors encompassing an individual's marketability. These impairments result in such extensive loss in body functioning that the individual is still unable to perform the full range of work required, even going beyond SGA (Substantial Gainful Activity), if such work would require a person to cope with changes given the turmoil existing inside the person.

2.2. Criteria for Anxiety Disorders as a Disability

In the questionnaire, validating the impact of anxiety, including its influence on other relevant bodily or mental functions, insomnia and issues related to immune relaxation are common. This falls under the category of symptom management and sustained performance. The anxiety itself can hinder physical or mental therapy. The use of an ergonomic assessment can demonstrate that anxiety directly contributes to the development of insomnia or pain that interferes with rehabilitation. Just like with disability discrimination judgments, anxiety and its persistent effects must meet the aforementioned accepted analyses. The latter requires that the societal understanding of anxiety as a fixed state must be operational. A claim must be defined based on its relevance to specific judgments. Society as a whole may provide dental presumption and therapy for a state of anxiety, but in order to be classified as a disability, the state of anxiety must be so severe that treatment is necessary.

To be considered a disability under specific criteria, anxiety must meet certain criteria. In non-criterion instructions, Social Security says it is "recognizing the potential deleterious effects of intense anxiety problems on a person's quality of life." Additionally, prerequisites for general anxiety syndrome state, "we assess this problem not only based on its influence on your ability to perform physical, psychological, and job-related activities, but also on your ability to adapt to changes in your daily life. This includes problems with managing your household, conflicts within your family, disruptions in social interactions, and how to perform tasks independently. These will be assessed in a separate domain if they occur." Given our focus on counseling for those with anxiety disorders, Social Security equipment must be able to address broader anxiety issues and not just the details.

2.2. Criteria for Anxiety Disorders

3. Social Security Disability Benefits

Who Determines if I am Disabled: The local Social Security Office or local hospital or doctor's office where you live are where you can visit or make appointments to complete disability paperwork. The Social Security Administration determines your eligibility. To succeed, you must prove: a) You can show evidence of diagnosed anxiety disorder symptoms, the severity, and the duration of the symptoms. There will also be questions about your social life, what symptoms you have, your ability to work doing everyday activities, and what treatments you have tried. b) Proof that you are only limited to completing sedentary activities. If you are not sedentary and disabled, you will be asked if there are other things you can do with your physical and mental limitations. To determine the work you can do is based on age, education, and work experience.

How to Apply: The fastest and easiest way to apply is through the Social Security Administration's website. Applying through the website will save time, is easy to navigate, and you can draft and make changes to the application before it is submitted. Visit the Social Security Administration's website to apply for benefits. The site also has accessible information and tutorials in American Sign Language. If you have questions, you can talk to representatives who will help you without leaving your home through a tablet, smartphone, or a computer.

3) Low-income Subsidy (LIS) "Extra Help" - for individuals with limited income and resources to pay for the costs of prescription drugs. To qualify, an applicant's income should be $19,320 (single) or $32,800 (married). The value of the applicant's resources should be $14,790 (single) or $29,520 (married).

2) Supplemental Security Income (SSI) - also pays out monthly to children or adults who are disabled or blind for individuals if they meet the financial limits set by the Social Security Administration.

1) Social Security Disability Insurance (SSDI) - based on your parents' or your "credits" for work, and you must be "disabled" and limited in how you can work. Your full monthly benefits begin after a trial work period of nine months showing income and continue until you show you can do "substantial work."

3.1. Types of Benefits Available

In summary, if a person with a disability such as an anxiety disorder who also makes very little money and is unable to work, they may receive a combination of SSDI and SSI benefits, particularly if they have legally eligible children or spouses. If a person has a disability but needs to pursue education before returning to work, they are eligible to receive SSDI only. SSDI will continue to be made available to individuals if the government decides they can no longer work due to medical conditions regardless of earned income levels and available resources. In order to receive support from the government, qualified individuals must undergo an income and resource breakdown to figure out which of the two programs is best for them. This may be useful for individuals with disabilities who want to apply for federal support themselves, as they can review their potential choices.

There are two types of disability support that a disabled individual can receive under the Social Security framework: Supplemental Security Income (SSI) and Social Security Disability Insurance (SSDI). SSDI is funded by the Social Security system through general fund taxes and is managed by the federal government. Its primary purpose is to provide benefits to disabled individuals and their families. A person's impairment needs to be included in a list of qualified medical conditions, which include a legitimized anxiety disorder, phobias, panic attacks, and agoraphobia, as well as depression. SSI, contrarily, is run by the Social Security Administration (SSA). It provides monthly payments to eligible people who are either 65 and older, blind, or disabled and have very low income and limited resources. SSI benefits are also available to applicants who are statutorily blind or visually impaired.

3.2. Application Process and Eligibility Criteria

To qualify for benefits: You must have worked in jobs covered by Social Security. You must have a medical disability that meets Social Security's definition of disability. The definition of disability under Social Security is different from other programs. Social Security pays only for total disability and does not pay for partial or short-term disability. Orthopedic and mental disorders, including anxiety, are listed in the Social Security Administration (SSA) "blue book" for consideration. But for a wide range of other disorders such as substance abuse and crime, schizoaffective disorder, and autistic syndrome disorder, it is unclear what the SSA policy is. For individuals aged 18 or over, they can be awarded benefits if they meet SSA's definition of disability. Being granted benefits enables an individual to receive treatment for their condition and prescription insurance. However, benefits do not include cash payouts for their disabled condition.

The application process to receive Social Security disability benefits begins with the applicant proving that they meet the eligibility criteria. The Social Security Administration (SSA) assessment of applications for disability benefits is based on a variety of demographic and eligibility factors. Firstly, applicants must be under the age of 65 due to being a compulsory retiree or over 65 and not being eligible for retirement cash due to their lack of insured status. Little attention is given to the applicant's education, although it is a compulsory field in the application process and has no bearing on your eligibility to receive disability. It is crucial that your illness is acknowledged as being a qualifying disability as the SSA does not pay benefits on impairments that affect less than 12 months. The benefit payments through this program only begin once the applicant has not carried out a 'substantial gainful activity' (SGA) in at least 30 consecutive days. An application has to be submitted within 60 days from the last day worked. Hereafter, the applicant can be granted a brief EDP initiation period of 17 months as the first day of the month of disability. Applications reaching 65+ are awarded five months disability up to the day of attainment.

4. Workplace Accommodations for Individuals with Anxiety

It is important to tailor reasonable accommodations to each person's unique needs based on his or her functional limitations. With that in in mind, the Job Accommodation Network has provided suggestions for accommodating employees with various types of anxiety disorders. An example of the types of reasonable accommodations that have been suggested for employees with a diagnosed anxiety disorder is as follows. For an employee with a generalized anxiety disorder and panic attacks, it may be an effective accommodation for an employer to institute flexible scheduling for the employee, granting him or her leave for medical treatments, when needed, without termination of employment due to excessive absences. This is just one example and it is important for employers to tailor accommodations to each individual employee.

The ADA has a clear definition of which services are considered reasonable to expect employers to provide. Reasonable accommodations are changes or modifications to the rules, policies, practices, and physical structure of the worksite, to provide equal access to job opportunities for individuals with a wide range of disabilities. An accommodation is not considered reasonable if it would impose an "undue hardship" on the employer. These concerns are generally defined as either causing significant financial stress or creating a direct threat to the health and safety of employees, customers, or the overall public.

The federal government has stepped in to provide guidance to employers when it comes to employing individuals with disabilities, including those with anxiety disorders. The Americans with Disabilities Act of 1990 (ADA) requires that employers covered by the law provide reasonable accommodations to qualified employees with disabilities, unless doing so would pose an undue hardship on the employer. Since a covered employer cannot employ an individual with a disability if that individual is unable to perform the essential functions of the job, the ADA makes it illegal to discriminate against a qualified individual with a disability who is able to perform unmodified job duties.

4.1. Reasonable Accommodations under the Americans with Disabilities Act

Having recognized that requested accommodations may actually be necessary under an expansive definition of the requirements of the ADA, it is imperative next to ask what kind of strategies employers should pursue in considering these requests for reasonable accommodations for individuals with anxiety disorders. A first principle places the analysis at the employee level, that is, an individual who believes that she is affected by an anxiety disorder and has encountered a work-related problem because of the symptoms of the disorder should consider asking for a reasonable accommodation. At this level, individuals who meet the above criteria should also document the disability, the accommodation, and the connection between the two.

A less ambivalent aspect of the ADA is the requirement of employers to provide employees who have disabilities with "reasonable accommodations." A reasonable accommodation is defined as "any change in the work environment or in the way things are customarily done that enables a person with a disability to enjoy equal employment opportunities." An employer is explicitly not required to provide a requested accommodation that is not reasonable or that would create "undue hardship" for the employer. If an individual provides adequate documentation of a disabling anxiety disorder and the need for a reasonable accommodation, it is at this point that the ADA takes on the task of recognizing both the potential for stigma experienced by the employee to the advantage of the employer as a strategic actor but also the independent physiological impact that anxiety disorders can have on the body. In the case of reasonable accommodations, "needed adjustments not only counteracted the strain of subordinating the disclosure of a stigmatized identity to strategic reward maximization, they also minimized the physical manifestations of the anxiety disorder."

4.1. Reasonable accommodations under the Americans with Disabilities Act

4.2. Examples of Accommodations for Anxiety Disorders

Cancel leave, or the contingency of such, and attend make up or virtual therapy. Adjusting work schedules, including having—and following—specific beginning and ending time for one's work day and/or week, and providing enough advance notice of changes in schedules and of meetings. Allowing phone calls at work that permit support persons to provide guidance when tasks are challenging. Shortened work day. Allowing regular breaks. A choice of computer-based or other ways to present documents or learning materials, including online texts/reading. A choice of email or hard copy for receiving workplace news. If you have employer-provided insurance, adding leave for additional medications. Permitting food at work in anticipation of extended leave for cognitive (non-trigger) medications needed in the afternoon. Providing a list of "the day's work".

If human rights and justice are to have any meaning, support should be provided for individuals with anxiety or other psychiatric diagnoses, both in seeking employment, if they desire, and in the workplace. This can be done through social security benefits and by requiring that employers provide the appropriate accommodations for all individuals, regardless of any health-related condition. Accommodations can be quite simple and not cost a great amount, financially or administratively, and can be incredibly effective. When specific accommodations are suggested—whether due to requests from individuals or frontline service providers to policy analysts and think-tanks and others creating resources for workplaces—they are often related to physical barriers such as those due to other health conditions or injuries, sensory disabilities, and even learning and intellectual differences, rather than for psychiatric and other cognitive processing differences and difficulties.

5. Support Services for Individuals with Anxiety

The Autism Society hosts a number of national and local programs for family support. Parents and family members of children with anxiety and depression can access these support groups. Many "spa-therapy" or in-house/day-treatment programs and camps exist for children and adolescents with anxiety who are battling social skills challenges, as do outpatient opportunity groups. There may be meetings, luncheon presentations, and conferences on anxiety. Yet, the American Counseling Association suggests that an anxiety support group should: be facilitated by a professional behavioral health clinician who is skilled in leading groups; require an intake interview with one or more of the anxiety group leaders to determine appropriateness for the group; have an appropriate length of time for a member to be involved (most assure several months); and have a written, educational and educational group curriculum. Given the broad availability and range of support services available for individuals with anxiety, it is increasingly understood that addressing anxiety must be all-encompassing; in order to be overcome, anxiety must be addressed systemically and consistently.

There are numerous support services that are available for individuals with anxiety. The primary category centers around therapeutic treatments provided by psychologists, mental health clinicians, and even primary care physicians. This can include every mode of treatment – from counseling to medications to direct intervention protocols such as Cognitive Behavior Therapy, and beyond. In so-called "non-clinical settings," numerous support services may be offered, including counseling via clergy or service members in religious denominations and not-for-profit organizations such as the United Way. Community support services often provide information resources, support, education, and training.

5.1. Therapeutic Interventions and Counseling

Cognitive-behavioral therapy is the most highly recommended therapeutic intervention for individuals with anxiety disorders. The basic assumption of CBT is that some distressing conditions result from inappropriate ways of thinking and behaving. CBT helps individuals to change these patterns. Cognitive-behavioral therapy consists of two main components: cognitive therapy and behavioral therapy, which are often used in conjunction with each other to achieve more effective outcomes. Cognitive therapy helps individuals to develop more comforting and adaptive ways of thinking. In other words, it assists the individual to "think differently." Cognitive therapy helps individuals to identify the irrational beliefs and misconstrued thought processes that happen as a result of anxiety and that perpetuate the anxiety.

5.1.1. Cognitive-Behavioral Therapy (CBT)

The management of anxiety disorders often includes some course of therapeutic intervention to assist an individual in gaining insight into the nature of their disorder, understanding their symptoms, and developing effective strategies for managing their condition. Therapeutic interventions take many forms, with different primary goals. In this section, we will briefly describe some of the recognized therapeutic options for individuals with anxiety disorders. This will allow you to gain a basic understanding of the different treatment options available to individuals, thus allowing you to make an informed decision about what intervention may be most useful for you.

5.1. Therapeutic Interventions and Counseling

5.2. Community Resources and Support Groups

Although we, as a society, have a long way to go before non-mental-ill people develop an accurate understanding of what it is like to have a mental illness, there has been a surge in attention lately on the topic of anxiety for several reasons. This increased awareness and acceptance can be useful for people with anxiety as it helps to make clear to them that they are not alone. In addition to the advice and emotional support from others, there are also many private mental health professionals accessible who can help with therapy, medication, or both for various types and levels of anxiety. Experts disagree on the quality and generalizability of studies on therapy for panic attacks or agoraphobia, but a common belief is that support group treatment, in particular, can help people become more capable and hopeful. However, it can be very hard for a person with anxiety to get help for it and to actually travel to help, especially if it is in an unfamiliar location.

Communities sometimes have networks or support groups for people with anxiety disorders or, more generally, for people with mental health issues. These can be one way to ensure that people with anxiety, who may be embarrassed to share their fears with friends or families who are neurotypical, can still find support over shared challenges. Members of the group will have likely shared advice on the best sympathetic doctors or courses of treatment based on their experiences and helped each other out in a variety of other ways. People who work with or for these groups may also have good general advice about local resources for disability or accommodations, including how to navigate the process to get them. Support members might be good sources of practical as well as emotional support.

6. Conclusion and Future Directions

Third, we need to increase specific services and develop appropriate interventions and policies. Perhaps this may be done by re-evaluating the levels at which the regulatory guiding systems of disability support, such as colleges and universities, consider accessibility-related accommodations and services for individuals who are temporarily or situationally at risk of inappropriate incapacitation from realistic anxiety that results from normal but often inherently anxiety-provoking experiences, like testing. What we do about this is an open question - maybe one we'll address in conclusion. Research is also needed on this. More structural work is also necessary, including collecting and analyzing complaints. Finally, we must train healthcare providers in the diagnosis and management of anxiety. This could lead to a richer discussion of who is "disabled enough" to warrant accommodations, particularly as discussed by Ettner et al. 2015, including both institutional and individual factors, particularly as anxiety disorders overlap with population-level "normal" affect.

Ultimately, anxiety and disability are constantly in tension, but they are not mutually exclusive. Both individual health and public health scholars must consider the ways in which anxiety is categorized as an impairment that needs accommodations or supports as outlined under the ADA. Our overview of these systems led to three key insights: First, the public health and clinical understandings of anxiety are tricky and conflictual. Further research is sorely needed. Second, many forms of support that are possible in public settings already exist (e.g., bathroom accommodations, testing centers without chairs). However, do these need to be explicitly designed with the specific mental health condition in mind in order to be more tailorable? Do we need to conduct more research that tailors each potential systems level or individualized strategies to specific forms of disabilities or latter, specific anxiety diagnoses (e.g., specific panic disorders) to assess the limits of responses that also help folks living with mostly debilitating anxiety disorders find a little algorithmic normalcy? We think the answer to this is certainly "yes".

An Examination of Anxiety Disorders and Disability Benefits

1. Introduction to Anxiety Disorders and Disability Benefits

Establishing eligibility for disability benefits is not only a multifaceted process but an extensive one. The majority of applicants for DSP receive multiple denials of their claim before they are approved for benefits. What is especially notable is that mental health claims for DSP are initially denied at a higher rate compared to all other disability categories while suffering more frequent multiple initial denials. Individuals who have their disability claims denied are forced to fight for the benefits that they qualify for through the Social Security Appeals Process in order to have their case reviewed. Among these individuals are more than 2.2 million Americans suffering from a mental disorder with more than half qualifying as a person affected by an anxiety disorder.

Anxiety disorders can be severely debilitating, to the point where individuals are unable to leave their homes for work, engage in tasks that include interactions with the public, or cope with the pressures and demands of a workplace setting. With certain jobs making these factors essential for employment, individuals affected by severe anxiety are often precluded from participating in these opportunities. Some individuals with anxiety disorders apply for Disability Support Pension (DSP) through the Social Security Administration (SSA) to receive government aid because they are unable to work; however, the process of applying for disability benefits is a very competitive and consuming one. One should consider an understanding of how anxiety disorders are currently represented in the array of available mental disorder listings used in the determination of eligibility for DSP and the processes involved in applying for these benefits, such as completing a residual functional capacity, an inability assessment that lists job-related tasks, an impairment assessment that lists symptoms of mental disorders, and functional assessment that determines whether an individual can work not only in their previous job but also in any other job that exists in significant numbers.

2. Types of Anxiety Disorders

• Generalized Anxiety Disorder (GAD) - Excessive worry concerning events and activities, physical symptoms, and potential dangers; anxiety that lasts for at least 6 months. • Panic Disorder is characterized by the occurrence of panic attacks, or unexpected rushes of terror combined with a constellation of symptoms, including shortness of breath, dizziness, and anxiety about loss of control or impending death. Panic disorder is often complicated by the development of agoraphobia, in which the person becomes afraid to leave the security of the home. • Social anxiety disorder (or social phobia) - Severe worry about not only performance, but also everyday activities when others are watching, presenting a deep fear of humiliation. Both situations are avoided, or endured with fear. • Specific phobia - Overwhelming fear of objects or situations; marked and excessive fear and anxiety about a specific object or situation; exposure to the phobic stimulus almost invariably provokes an immediate anxiety response, which may take the form of a situationally bound or situationally predisposed panic attack. • Obsessive-compulsive disorder (OCD) - Persistent, unwanted fears (obsessions) that trigger anxiety or the repetitive behaviors that are driven by the obsessive fears (compulsions); clients realize the thoughts are a product of their mind and are not based in reality, but are unable to stop them. • Post-traumatic stress disorder (PTSD) - Traumatic events such as seeing or witnessing a traumatic event, sexual assault, warfare, or an accident; often results in vivid "flashbacks" that involve disturbing memories and images of the traumatic event, and intense physical and emotional distress.

An anxiety disorder is a psychiatric condition that produces uncontrolled fear, worry, or stress with severe and relentless symptoms that may interfere with a person's daily life. The major types of anxiety disorders are summarized in the American Psychiatric Association (APA) Diagnostic and Statistical Manual of Mental Disorders (DSM-5). Criteria for diagnosis are as follows:

2.1. Generalized Anxiety Disorder (GAD)

People diagnosed with generalized anxiety disorder frequently have co-occurring psychiatric illnesses, such as mood and psychotic disorders, and anxiety disorders, such as panic attacks, social anxiety, and apparent anxiety attacks. A range of cognitive and behavioral structured psychotherapies for the treatment of general practitioners (CBT) can prove effective in serving people with GAD. While some clinicians will suggest antidepressant therapy as the primary care for thousands of unrelated people with generalized anxiety disorder in therapy, studies have shown that the best approach is medication management alone. As a result, some enhancements have been made to standard medical therapy. Regardless, treatment efficacy can be determined by whether the consumer experiences minimal or no discomfort, irrespective of their original approach to care. Remember: having GAD does not automatically qualify for SSDI or SSI benefits. If, for example, you own a small coffee shop and have GAD, your disability claim is likely to be denied because coffee shop owners do not qualify for SSI or SSDI benefits.

Effectively applying for federal disability benefits for individuals with anxiety disorders necessitates an understanding of the disorder's characteristics, symptoms, and overall impact on development. Generalized anxiety disorder (GAD) is the most prevalent of all anxiety disorders. In clinical settings, it affects about 5% of people in one year. It is characterized by excessive and possibly unrealistic anxiety and concern about at least two different life situations, for a considerable time, several months. In comparison to those of the same age, the worrying can be amplified by physical or somatic symptoms, such as muscular tension, tiredness, or sleeping problems.

2.2. Panic Disorder

Twenty percent of American soldiers have been diagnosed with panic disorder, with most also being diagnosed with other anxiety and/or mental disorders (Dupre, 2011). Awareness of panic disorder has grown in recent years, and new drugs have been developed to treat it. It is beginning to have implications in the disability arena, as individuals who present with panic disorder are either not being granted disability benefits, have had their current advantage decreased, or have been required to go back to work as a result of the disorder (Gay, 2018). Clearly, panic disorder has a major impact on the ability to work and function. What is not clear is to what extent the disorder is responsible for the amount of anxiety. Panic disorder does not have to play a role in the denial of disability benefits, since people may yet meet the criteria for P&T advantages due to another medical condition. In your help with getting benefits, you will have to work with your incumbent supervisor before getting your compensation.

Panic disorder, according to the DSM-5 (APA, 2013), is a severe and recurrent panic attack coupled with worrisome and daunting thoughts or real-time behavioral changes as well as marked alterations in thinking or behavior (Benton, 2016). Symptoms can include chest pains, nausea, dizziness, feelings of detachment, feelings of sweating or chills, numbness or tingling, a trembling or quivering sensation, increased heart rates, chest pains, excessive thoughts of collapsing or dying, fears of losing control, as well as feeling an imminent peril or danger (Smith, 2016).

A person with panic disorder may avoid locations or events that might trigger attacks since panic attacks are unpredictable, and as such, it is impossible to understand when they will happen. Panic attacks also have the consequence of debilitating individuals both physically and emotionally for a variable amount of time (Smith, 2016).

2.3. Social Anxiety Disorder

Possible Impairment Estimated Worldwide, approximately 12% of individuals will experience social anxiety disorder at some time in their lifetime. It is the third most common psychological disorder in the United States. The typical age of onset is 13 years old. Symptoms include intense fear that does not subside, rather it worsens over time, so it is important to begin treatment at the first signs of anxiety. Physicians might first offer anxiolytics with cognitive therapy before using other therapy. Other effective treatments may include selective serotonin reuptake inhibitors (SSRIs) or other antianxiety agents, psychotherapy groups to offer social skill building, or general counseling. As more categories of social anxiety disorder treatment are tried, the opportunities for receiving approval for Social Security Disability benefits increases. Consequently, social anxiety disorder is usually most often experienced by individuals 13 years old and older, and it begins to interfere with their daily activities.

Social anxiety disorder (SAD) is characterized by significant anxiety when it comes to social settings and activities. Individuals might then isolate themselves or experience problems in social settings. Social anxiety disorder entails intense fear of public embarrassment or scrutiny. It could even be a fear of causing oneself embarrassment in front of others. Physical symptoms of social anxiety disorder can include symptoms of panic such as heart palpitations, blushing, sweating, and dizziness. Individuals diagnosed with social anxiety disorder may also have body dysmorphic disorder, panic disorder, obsessive-compulsive disorder, and severe depression.

2.4. Specific Phobias

Each specific phobia directly implicates either mobility or personal safety or both. The phobias address wild animals, plants, the like, and modern machines: dogs, insects, snakes, mice, spiders, rats, cats, birds, other animals, bees, ants, roaches, trees, storm winds, deep ocean waters, bad weather, other natural environments, driving cars, riding as a passenger in a car, other vehicles, operating public transit vehicles, heights, escalators, elevators, closed places, planes, getting-to-a-health-care-professional scenes, and getting blood tests. Phobia we define as a disabling illness. Some legal cases have upheld restrictions imposed by specific phobias. However, evidence regarding the occupational and social consequences of having a specific phobia is typically excluding. This can often include evidence concerning the phobia's occupational implications. Anxiety disorders can now be proven because reactivity is one symptom in all the anxiety disorders. Most often the appropriate evidence helps purport Uncle Sam's right to deny a claimant's claim for benefits. The result can be claimant difficulty documenting occupational consequences of his concern.

Unrealistic fear or anxiety triggered by the presence or anticipation of a specific object or situation is the defining characteristic of each specific phobia in the DSM-5's list of phobias. What defines a specific phobia is currently the same as what defined it in the DSM-III except for two revisions. First, in the DSM-III, specific phobias were labeled simple phobias, a term that was replaced in the

DSM-IV and DSM-5 with the current DSM-III term. Second, the DSM-5's list of specific phobias is those the DSM-III termed slight, mild, and moderate specified. Differentiating a specific phobia is separation of fear of the object from risk the object presents (doctrine of double apprehension).

2.5. Obsessive-Compulsive Disorder (OCD)

OCD is a common disorder and causes distress in many individuals in the workplace. However, obtaining disability allowance can be very hard for people with the condition.

Secondly, a broad range of abilities outside of attention and concentration are required for different types of work. Interpersonal skills are needed for jobs requiring teamwork, customer relations, or supervision. OCD often causes people to question their own actions and motives and be hyper-critical of themselves. It is not hard to see that jobs requiring a very high level of vocational skill, i.e. where there is little or no room for error, may be hard for someone with this illness. There is a vicious cycle of anxiety surrounding work primed by the stress of getting and keeping a job. The vulnerable job market makes anxious people even more critical of their own performance, leading to more anxiety, leading to more self-doubt.

OCD can increase disability in two main ways. First, inefficiency or decreased productivity while at work can occur. This is because people with OCD experience a decrease in attention and an increase in their time in performing rituals. Additionally, psychiatric research often links OCD and mood disorders. People with OCD are more likely to experience depression, anxiety, other anxiety disorders, and alcohol abuse compared to the rest of the population. These additional psychiatric symptoms can make it even harder to concentrate at work.

Obsessive thoughts are ones that constantly intrude upon an individual's consciousness. They cause the sufferer to feel a high level of anxiety. Rituals or compulsions are performed to neutralize or decrease that anxiety. These compulsions can be either mental or physical. While OCD is sometimes thought of as only hand washing or making sure the door is locked, it impacts nearly every aspect of an individual's life including work and relationships.

Obsessive-Compulsive Disorder (OCD) is a common, chronic mental illness. When most people think of OCD, they picture someone vigorously washing their hands or a compulsive hoarder. However, real OCD is much more than that. OCD's symptoms can be particularly unique to each individual, but recurrent unwanted thoughts and rituals constitute the two primary symptoms of OCD.

2.6. Post-Traumatic Stress Disorder (PTSD)

Post-traumatic stress disorder often occurs with other anxiety disorders, depression, substance abuse, or somatization disorder. PTSD, when it occurs in conjunction with other conditions, tends to be more chronic and less amenable to treatment. It is common for a person to experience acute stress disorder immediately following a trauma and later develop PTSD. Entry criteria for PTSD in the DSM-IV require exposure to a traumatic event, with the individual experiencing symptoms in three functional areas: hyperarousal, re-experiencing, and avoidance. Impairment in social and occupational areas of functioning is also present. Triggers for this disorder include war, rape, natural disasters, hostage situations, and any other unjustifiable personal assault. PTSD restricts the ability of an individual to function normally. Research has shown that about one-third of persons with PTSD had symptoms after 10 years. The major causes of work-related PTSD are related to catastrophic accidents, participation in wartime activities, and having experienced crime.

PTSD is a fear-related disorder triggered by a real or imagined traumatic or life-threatening event in the individual. The individual's ability to function is affected as it involves the cognitive processing or memory of the event. The condition results in a diminished interest in previously enjoyed activities. There may also be an avoidance of activities that remind the individual of the event. Recurrent images or thoughts of the event may intrude the consciousness of the individual, and the individual may relive some aspect of the trauma. The individual may experience nightmares or flashbacks, which can occur suddenly and without any apparent trigger. The individual is chronically "on edge," may have problems sleeping, and may have difficulty relating to others.

3. Criteria for Qualifying for Disability Benefits

Individuals who apply for Social Security disability benefits are likely to wonder what qualifies someone as disabled. As this article explains, functional capacity is evaluated and mental limitations are considered. Also, several factors related to the functional assessment. One of the factors listed is mental limitations resulting from mental health issues such as anxiety. Although functional capacity is assessed in a consultative examination (CE) that results in a report, there is no reference to the actual performance levels on record indicating that the consulting physician examined an explanation of how the subject's insufficient function relates to a specific aspect of work. Records also do not refer to the requirements of the SSA's medical equivalence to listings. This suggests that the abysmal function reported in the case file may have made for compelling evidence of medical equivalence.

The Social Security Administration (SSA) has a list of criteria that a person needs to meet to qualify for Social Security Disability Insurance (SSDI) and Supplemental Security Income (SSI) benefits. The SSA looks at the effect of the symptoms that the applicant has. When listing the factors he considers when deciding a case, a hearing office director with the SSA indicated that the evaluator may rate the severity of such mental conditions as anxiety primarily on the basis of their functional effect. The Mental Residual Functional Capacity (RFC) assessment rates a person's mental functional capacity on the basis of his abilities in making occupational adaptations. Examiners believe that a person's functioning is probably not the same as his ability to manage most basic work situations.

3.1. Social Security Administration (SSA) Guidelines

Applicants who have a diagnosis of, or a condition with symptoms of, an anxiety disorder are therefore advised to document their case as accurately and thoroughly as possible. For the SSA, eligibility for disability benefits based on either an application for Social Security Disability Insurance (SSDI) benefits or Supplemental Security Income (SSI) benefits will hinge on the degree to which one's anxiety is found to limit or impair the ability to complete subpart B or C criteria of the 12.06 listing for mental disorders. One will also need to supply additional documentation to prove that he or she meets the requirements within this listing. If at any time during the process of proving one's anxiety was present, even untreated, the SSA may award SSI benefits on a medical-vocational allowance basis as employees will examine one's Residual Functional Capacity (RFC) to make sure he or she can return to some type of gainful employment.

While the law does require that the Social Security Administration (SSA) develop guidelines for people who demonstrate psychological or mental impairments, it does not single out contemplation of those individuals with anxiety or other mood disorders. Instead, the law requires the SSA to use standardized criteria in the determination of all disability applications, including a cross-cutting emphasis that the SSA added in June of 2009, directing its adjudicators to examine the effect of any and all impairments on an applicant's ability to work by using the agency's 12.00 Listing of Impairments.

3.2. Mental Residual Functional Capacity (RFC) Assessment

The mental RFC assessment also provides the SSA with an idea of how a claimant's mental functioning can be affected by physical, social, and environmental limitations. In order to determine if a person's mental disorder(s) is sick enough to interfere with that person's employment, SSA employees can apply the mental RFC assessment in conjunction with a physical RFC, if that applies. The mental RFC used in the social security evaluation process can indicate the need for services for a person with severe mental illness. Information from the SSA's IRP can assist clinicians in advocating for their client in the process of receiving an appropriate mental RFC. A client can apply for mental health services at the Social Security Disability Advocate Program (DAP).

Mental Residual Functional Capacity (RFC) Assessment. The RFC assessment used by the Social Security Administration allows hearing officers at the initial, hearing, and Appeals Council stages of the disability claim process to evaluate a person's disorder-related impairments. The experts use the International Classification of Functioning, Disability and Health - a functional coding system developed by the World Health Organization - to guide them in defining limitations for persons at the first, second, third, fourth, and fifth percentile of functioning. This assessment is multisystemic and addresses 36 mental functions across five life areas: activities of daily living, social functioning, concentration, persistence, and pace; deterioration of work settings; and episodes of decompensation. Disability claims based on mental health disorders can be found not disabled if a person has a minimal choice of jobs under this multisystemic approach. The RFC assessment assists the SSA to determine what, if any, work a claimant is able to do with his or her mental disorder(s).

4. Types of Disability Benefits

Another informational article offers an overview of Social Security disability benefits for people with anxiety disorders for those who want an overview of the process and various benefits. An article also collectively examines in great detail every part of the disability benefit process including the initial application, the primary application, the appeal to an administrative law judge, and federal court appeals. An additional article specifically details SSI. It includes application procedures and rules of eligibility, but it takes a more detailed look into income and assets to allow a more complete overview of the application and application process, thus offering a great way to get an overview to those dealing specifically with SSI.

Many people do not know the complexities of Social Security disability benefits, and disability benefits may be more varied than one may suppose. Disability benefits for those with anxiety disorders come in two primary types: Social Security Disability Insurance (SSDI) and Supplemental Security Income (SSI). In order to qualify for SSDI, a person must have an anxiety disorder along with other serious disabilities, and she must have been previously employed and paid taxes into Social Security. SSI benefits, on the other hand, are for disabled individuals who do not have an extensive employment history. These benefits vary, so many articles concentrate on the circumstances and benefits of a particular type of benefit. For example, one informational article offers insights to a particular group: the most common cause is listing 12.06 on the anxiety disorder listing. In order to qualify for benefits under the listing, an individual must meet the criteria of the listing.

The amount of monthly disability benefits to which a claimant may be entitled is determined by his or her work history and specifically by his or her average indexed monthly earnings (AIME). An SSDI beneficiary's spouse and children may also be eligible to receive benefits based on the beneficiary's work record. After receiving disability benefits for two years, SSDI recipients who meet Social Security's definition of disabled will qualify for Medicare, which provides access to doctors and hospitals at reduced rates. In recent years, some policymakers and commentators have expressed concerns over the SSDI application process, with particular focus on high denial rates. As one critic notes, less than 5 percent of SSDI applicants are approved at the first step of the application process, and only 36 percent are approved at the appeals level. Failed applicants can wait years to have their cases resolved, and the appeals process may require the assistance of an attorney. In the sections that follow, we describe some of the features of the SSDI application process that may be particularly challenging for people with anxiety disorders and other disabilities.

Social Security Disability Insurance (SSDI) provides financial support to people who have a severe anxiety disorder and who have worked and paid into Social Security for enough years to qualify for disability benefits. Eligibility for SSDI depends largely on the claimant's work history. In order to qualify, an applicant must have worked a certain number of years - out of the 10 years before applying for benefits - and must have worked 5 out of 10 of the years before becoming disabled (the specific amount of work history required to qualify for benefits depends on the claimant's age). In addition, an applicant must have a medical condition that meets the Social Security Administration's definition of disability. Anxiety disorders that may qualify for disability benefits include generalized anxiety disorder, panic disorder, agoraphobia, and social anxiety disorder, as well as other mental health disorders such as depression and bipolar disorder.

4.1. Social Security Disability Insurance (SSDI)

4.2. Supplemental Security Income (SSI)

The purpose of the SSI program is to provide a minimum income to individuals and married couples who are blind or disabled or are aged 65 or older and have very limited income and resources. To qualify for SSI, individuals must apply and be determined to be aged, blind, or disabled according to federal rules and requirements. The monthly payment varies up to the federal monthly maximum. In 2022, the monthly payment standard for an SSI individual is $841, and the monthly standard for a couple is $1,261. Individuals apply for SSI benefits at their local Social Security office and may apply online, in person, by mail, or by telephone. The initial application is reviewed by the local Social Security office, and then the application is sent to a state agency for an application for disability benefits. Many applicants are denied at the initial stage, and those who are denied can request to have their application reconsidered.

The Social Security Administration (SSA) administers several programs that provide resources to individuals with disabling anxiety disorders, including Supplemental Security Income (SSI). Established in 1972, SSI is critically important because, in contrast to Social Security Disability Insurance (SSDI), it does not require the individual to have a work history. SSI payments aid more than 8 million Americans who are disabled, blind, or elderly with low incomes. Adults and children who receive SSI are entitled to Medicaid benefits. In 2020, about 145,000 individuals with anxiety disorder diagnoses received SSI, which is 5% of new SSI allowances due to mental disorders.

5. Process of Applying for Disability Benefits

Whether or not the applicant is approved, the applicants have the right to appeal. The first stage of appeal is the same as the initial application stage. Following the reconsideration stage is the hearing process. At the hearing level, the applicant is entitled to an in-person administrative hearing with an administrative law judge (ALJ) who is not associated with the state or the Social Security Administration. At the hearing, the applicant has the right to be represented by an attorney and present witnesses. The ALJ also has the right, at his or her own discretion, to call a medical expert and/or a vocational expert. If, after going through the appeals process, the applicant is still denied benefits, he or she may file a civil action in the federal district court. While this process appears detailed and extensive, it is not nearly this easy.

The process for applying for disability benefits is notoriously difficult, often leaving those who need government help in the lurch. Initially, the applicant must fill out forms that detail their current and past medical history as well as a detailed list of employment and relevant education. From there, the office of Disability Determination allows a state agency to gather medical information. If the medical evidence gathered is not enough, the Disability Determination service is responsible for arranging a consultative medical examination (CME). The state agency will then make a decision based on the medical information gathered on whether or not the applicant is disabled. Every year from this step, 67 percent of adults with anxiety disorders see their application for Social Security benefits denied. For applicants with General Anxiety Disorder (GAD), panic disorder or depression, the denial rate is 81 percent.

Other things you may want to collect or discuss prior to filing an application include, but are not limited to, detailed home remedies and treatment for your conditions, a list of your job approvals and dates of same, and you will have to decide whether you want to add eligible beneficiaries or file for Medicare. If the claim is an SSI claim, the application may also include whether the claimant can work and how much, or about income received, in-kind help received, and living arrangements. For somebody with anxiety, it is important to document ways that the symptoms impact your ability to carry out activities of daily living. It is important to document physical symptoms that may accompany your anxiety, cognitive impairments, or panic attacks. A statement from friends or family about how the anxiety has impacted your life is also key. You also will need to discuss a complete list of medications and non-physician prescribed medications, if relevant. You will also need a list of mental health professionals, along with contact information, that you have sought treatment or been treated for your anxiety.

The first step in applying for disability is to submit an application for benefits with the Social Security Administration (SSA). You may fill out an application online, in person, over the phone, or by mail. During this step, you must provide personal information including, but not limited to: name, address, and phone number; the names, addresses, and phone numbers of any doctors, hospitals, medical professionals, clinics, labs, etc. that you have received any kind of treatment for your disability; your work history for the last 15 years, and information of any workers' compensation you are filing. Additionally, you must submit a complete Adult Disability Report and a complete Authorization to Disclose Information to the SSA.

Appeals for SSI and RSDI deferrals may be filed after 10 calendar days have gone by since the notice was given, excluding the date the denial notice was received. If the deadline for the appeal falls on a Saturday, Sunday, or a legal public holiday, the last day is a following Federal working day. Next in the appeals process, if after the reconsideration a claim is still denied or receives a determination, the claimant has 60 days to file a request for hearing before an administrative law judge. If again denied, the claimant has 60 days to appeal to the Social Security Appeals Council (in writing). The same process applies to both SSI and RSDI claimants. Individuals can appeal their denials if they do not understand the disability decision made, if they believe facts were not adequately presented concerning a claim and the health condition, if they believe additional relevant facts and evidence are available to support their claim, and if they believe the law was not correctly applied.

After the initial application period ends, the Social Security Administration will notify the claimant of the decision for their application. If an application is denied (which is not uncommon at this stage in the process), the individual has the right to appeal that decision. Individuals have 60 days from the date of the denial notice for the reconsideration or appeal. For individuals filing appeals concerning SSI and the RSDI, the claimant can appeal the denial online or fill out a "Request for Reconsideration" form. The appeals process appointment can be conducted over the phone, allowing individuals who experience anxiety leaving the house or other phobias face-to-face contact to plead their case from the comfort of home.

6. Other Types of Benefits and Accommodations

There are state mental health services available in every state and many local communities. Clinics, programs, and services provide a wide range of treatments and supports to help people with anxiety disorders continue to work and remain as independent as possible. The types of service a person with an anxiety disorder receives will depend on their need, diagnosis, and insurance plan. Treatment for anxiety disorders will include psychotherapy and medicines. Some clinics and programs also offer further treatments and recovery support, such as vocational rehabilitation and supported employment, respite services, peer support, supported housing, and social and recreational activities. These services can help restore emotional well-being. Overcoming your medical condition may also involve such recovery activities as finding an activity club to join, furthering your education, or getting job training to increase your income. They can also develop job-related skills if you are prepared to work. A variety of job-related services are available in many communities, including counseling, job placement assistance, and training.

In addition to Supplemental Security Income (SSI) and Social Security Disability Insurance (SSDI), there are also state benefits programs that provide individuals with anxiety disorders assistance. There are also other types of accommodations. Under the Americans with Disabilities

Act, individuals with anxiety disorders are required to be given reasonable accommodations by their employer. The accommodations must make it easier for the employee to apply for, perform, and enjoy the benefits of employment. Some examples include altering an employee's job responsibilities, making the employee's work schedule more flexible, decreasing the amount of work given to the employee, allowing the employee to be absent from work for doctor's appointments, and excusing the employee's occasional poor performance.

6.1. Reasonable Accommodations in the Workplace

Information contained herein should not be considered legal counsel. It is generally advisable to consult an attorney who can consider the particulars of a particular case. This list is meant to be illustrative and by no means provides a complete list of possible accommodations. Managers should initiate an interactive process with the affected employee to determine which reasonable accommodations are suitable for each particular situation.

* Flexible scheduling, breaks, and remote work options (e.g., telework) to attend medical appointments that individuals may not be able to schedule outside their work hours. * Accommodations for individuals who have physical symptoms that cause them to miss work (i.e. providing leave during periods of severe physical symptoms). * Environmental controls, such as noise machines, to reduce work-related stress. * Technology or software that prompts reminders to take work breaks or practice self-care. * A quiet workspace or conference room where individuals can go to relax.

Individuals with anxiety disorders may find the following reasonable accommodations helpful:

Individuals with anxiety disorders may require reasonable accommodations within the workplace due to their mental health condition(s) and/or symptoms. A reasonable accommodation is defined as modification(s) to a job position or employment process that enable a qualified individual with a disability to be considered for a job, perform the essential duties of a job, or to enjoy benefits, privileges, or services in all aspects of employment.

6.2. Mental Health Services and Resources

Psychology of anxiety and anxiety disorders, and a unique feature of this psychology is its impact. Much of the psychological research has focused on the aspects of the sufferer: trying to identify, define, and classify the disorder. In this foundation topic, we have investigated the impact of the anxiety disorders on the lives of those who have the condition, and how the National Mental Health Report for Australia summarizes the findings of a substantial body of such research. This research categorizes and reports on the use of a range of health and welfare services specifically suited to the treatment of adults with a variety of anxiety disorder diagnoses, including agoraphobia, panic disorder, and social phobia. Information on services provided by private mental health professionals, general field services, primary care settings, and emergency care services is highlighted, along with a summary of the key findings in this area that are discussed within the National Mental Health Report for Australia.

There are numerous services, treatments, and resources that anxiety disorder sufferers can access to manage their symptoms, including health professionals such as general and specialist doctors (such as a psychiatrist or clinical psychologist), private, public, and other alternative counseling or therapy services, and online and remote-based and e-health services. Additionally, various support networks and mental health programs have been set up for individuals with anxiety disorders, as well as their families, partners, and friends (if requested). A number of programs designed to train primary health care professionals in diagnosing and treating individuals with anxiety disorders are in place, as are associations and programs designed to educate, train, and support mental health service staff within anxiety disorder settings. While it is evident that there is a variety of anxiety disorder services available for people with anxiety disorders, many of these findings are located in specialist settings and exclude particular groups of anxious individuals that are not at the severe end of the spectrum. There is little information about how successful such programs are in treating anxiety disorders. It is important to note that there are over 300 references to "anxious" patients and over 100 references to "anxious" adults. However, none of these studies specifically mention adults or partners that are pension-age.

7. Conclusion and Recommendations

Based on this evidence, this essay recommends enhanced training for occupations such as physicians and other relevant professionals to better recognize the subjective constraints experienced by individuals with anxiety disorders and appreciate their unique circumstances with increased cultural competence. To this end, a semi-qualified or qualified clinician might be employed to recognize cases of subjective functional underperformance, commonly associated with anxiety disorders, in a medical committee capacity. It is recommended that the relevant legislation used to select candidates to receive requested social security checks should take into account the invisible functionality losses, social barriers, and practical analytical difficulties that applicants with anxiety disorders might be facing. It is also suggested that the relevant biology of anxiety disorders be included in relevant disability criteria to better reflect the nuances of what an individual with this disorder might be going through in terms of a diversity of possible interpretations of physical constraints on written medical evidence. If something is to be considered a tool to increase do-goodership in the disability assessment process, something similar to the affirmative-action processes in hiring opportunities could be considered to widen the proportion of vulnerable and marginalized individuals that receive requested requests for disability benefits.

The conclusion of this paper can be summarized in two points. Firstly, anxiety disorders are a type of mental disorder that might be difficult for a third party to observe and differentiate from stress, sadness, and other emotions, both qualitatively and quantitatively. Individuals suffering from anxiety disorders may experience life in complex or even terrifying ways that make it difficult for them to relate to their surroundings. Anxiety disorders pose invisible and subjective constraints in terms of loss of functionality, making them difficult to observe and gauge. In this essay, evidence was collected by asking key informants in the field of social security what types of professional evidence work best for selecting or excluding vulnerable candidates for a social security check. Additionally, it was not adequately addressed in legislation that acknowledges the needs of vulnerable individuals with anxiety disorders during the process of acquiring disability benefits.